Promoting person-centred care at the front line

Anthea Innes, Suzi Macpherson and Louise McCabe

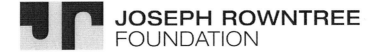

JOSEPH ROWNTREE
FOUNDATION

The **Joseph Rowntree Foundation** has supported this project as part of its programme of research and innovative development projects, which it hopes will be of value to policy makers, practitioners and service users. The facts presented and views expressed in this report are, however, those of the authors and not necessarily those of the Foundation.

Joseph Rowntree Foundation, The Homestead, 40 Water End, York YO30 6WP
Website: www.jrf.org.uk

About the authors

Dr Anthea Innes is Course Director of MSc Dementia Studies at the University of Stirling. Her research interests focus on health and social care for older people, including people with dementia. Dr Innes has authored a number of publications concerned with dementia and dementia care.

Dr Suzi Macpherson is a Lecturer in Social Policy at the University of Stirling. Her research interests focus on disability and social inclusion, promoting a social model perspective to support disabled people's inclusion.

Dr Louise McCabe is a Lecturer in Dementia Studies in the Department of Applied Social Science at the University of Stirling. Her research interests include social policy, health and social care practice and services for older people and people with dementia.

ISBN-13: 978 1 85935 451 3
ISBN-10: 1 85935 451 3

A pdf version of this publication is available from the JRF website (www.jrf.org.uk).

A CIP catalogue record for this report is available from the British Library.

Cover design by Adkins Design

Prepared and printed by:
York Publishing Services Ltd
64 Hallfield Road
Layerthorpe
York
YO31 7ZQ
Tel: 01904 430033   Fax: 01904 430868   Website: www.yps-publishing.co.uk

Further copies of this report, or any other JRF publication, can be obtained either from the JRF website (www.jrf.org.uk/bookshop/) or from our distributor, York Publishing Services Ltd, at the above address.

Contents

Acknowledgements vii

Executive summary viii

1 Introduction 1
Methods 2

2 Person-centred care 5
Person-centred care 5
Good-quality support/care 11
Working effectively with families 19
Conclusions 23

3 Perceptions of frontline work 25
Qualities of workers 25
Practical skills 28
Caring as a relationship 32
Value of care work 35
Conclusions 41

4 Systemic and organisational issues for frontline workers 43
Systemic issues 43
Management 48
Training 51
Recruitment 55
Conclusions 57

5 Conclusions and recommendations 59
Summary and conclusions 59
Recommendations 61

References 65

Appendix 1: Approach to reviewing the literature 74

Appendix 2: Pro forma for the literature review 77

**Appendix 3: Focus group schedule – frontline workers
(same topics used for service user focus group)** 78

ACKNOWLEDGEMENTS

First, we wish to thank the members of our advisory group for their support. Second, the service providers who helped us identify frontline workers and service users to include in our discussion groups and focus groups. Finally, our thanks go to all the frontline workers and service users who participated in the discussion groups and focus groups and who shared their experiences with us.

Executive Summary

This study is about the barriers and opportunities to the delivery of person-centred support/care by frontline workers. The study also included a consultation process with service users and frontline workers; this process reinforced the findings from the literature.

The project, based at the Department of Applied Social Science, University of Stirling, involved three key stages.

1 At the start of the study, four discussion groups were held in the central belt of Scotland: one with disabled people, one with older people, one with frontline workers in the social care sector and one with frontline workers in the health sector who were from and working with minority ethnic communities.

2 A literature review exploring the barriers and opportunities facing frontline workers in promoting person-centred care for older people, disabled people and workers and service users from minority ethnic groups.

3 Towards the end of the study, three focus groups were held: one in Northern England with frontline workers and two in Scotland, one with service users and one with frontline workers.

Findings

Person-centred care

This concept is used mainly in the older people literature, particularly in relation to dementia care.

Quality support/care

Although the term 'person-centred care' may not be used, there is a general consensus that person-centred or quality care is care that: is focused on clients/users; promotes independence and autonomy rather than control; involves services that are reliable and flexible and chosen by users; and tends to be offered by those working in a collaborative/team philosophy.

Working effectively with families

Listening to carers' and service users' views, which may be contradictory, can be difficult. Management of the relationship between frontline workers and family members can also be challenging. The importance of supporting family relationships is central to providing quality care and involves frontline workers engaging in skilled communication.

Qualities of frontline workers

Users identify personal characteristics – gender, ethnicity and cultural background – as important, in addition to personal qualities such as patience, compassion, sensitivity and empathy. Skills to help perform their role are also valued. All of these issues feed into the relationship between user and frontline worker, and are pivotal to experiences of good-quality/person-centred care/support.

Barriers to quality care

Barriers relate predominantly to bureaucratic structures and services being service, rather than user, led. Additional barriers to good-quality care for people from minority ethnic groups are: lack of information made available to minority communities hindering their access to services; lack of cultural understanding inherent in services offered; and language and communication difficulties.

Management, training, recruitment and retention

Management practices tend to overlook the importance of relationships between frontline workers and clients. A move towards increased managerialism and budget-led services constrains frontline workers who feel they receive little support from management in their day-to-day work.

Training opportunities are inequitable for different frontline workers. There is also a lack of consensus about the impact of training on practice.

Recruitment and retention of frontline workers is a key concern within the literature, with pay and conditions cited as factors in the difficulties the care sector is currently facing.

Value of frontline work

There is a general undervaluing of care work throughout society despite policy documents stating the value of such work. Users' views of frontline workers tend to be obscured by a focus on general aspects of service provision rather than on their roles specifically. Engagement with frontline workers' views tends to be limited to particular professional groups, for example, social workers.

Recommendations

There are four specific research topics that could be developed.

- A study to explore frontline workers' specific roles and the requirements of them by service users – focusing on gathering views from both frontline workers and service users. This would provide an alternative and more focused approach to the previous service-delivery approach that has dominated research.

- A study that engages directly with frontline workers to explore their motivations, satisfactions and frustrations in their role. In particular, directly focusing on the drivers and challenges facing frontline workers – investigating the diversity of frontline workers, related to the tasks they undertake within their role and their age, gender and ethnicity.

- Research is required to gather a richer picture of service users' views and experiences of frontline care and support. A more detailed understanding is needed of the potential divergences between different service users' requirements. This could help promote a better understanding of the complexity in delivering care and support packages in practice.

- A study that aims to understand how frontline workers navigate the often contradictory demands of policy and practice change and the needs of service users. This could potentially offer insights into the complexities of meeting professional requirements while also delivering a suitable care/support package to their clients.

There are four areas where further policy and practice work could be undertaken.

- A scoping study to gather information on what frontline workers and service users define as 'good-quality support'. This would both improve knowledge relating to the notion of 'good-quality support' and focus more directly on gathering the views of service users and frontline workers rather than managers and policy makers.

- A national mapping exercise to identify and record both innovative and best practice where these are taking place. This would, not only offer an opportunity to disseminate this information, but also encourage and promote quality frontline care and support.

- A consultation exercise with frontline workers on their training needs and how these could best be met offers one way of gathering workers' views on the knowledge gaps they identify as preventing them delivering high-quality care.

- Finally, with practice lagging well behind policy rhetoric and ideology, consultation with those at the grass roots (frontline workers, service users and voluntary sector organisations) could shed some light on the reason for the delays occurring in practice. They could also offer suggestions from the grass-roots perspective for how best to implement change. The voice of service users and frontline workers could also usefully be brought into policy discourse through this exercise.

1 INTRODUCTION

Independent living has been promoted for disabled people and older people through the NHS and Community Care Act 1990 and the Direct Payments (Community Care) Act 1996 (Department of Health, 2004; Scottish Executive, 2004a). The development of National Care Standards for Scotland (Scottish Executive, 2004b) and the National Minimum Standards for care developed in England (National Care Standards Commission, 2004) both stress the need to recognise culturally appropriate service delivery for users of community and residential care services, acknowledging the need for user involvement in the delivery of community care services. These policy developments highlight the importance of a more 'person-centred' approach within community care services. Within this framework, however, little attention has been given to the role played by frontline workers in limiting, facilitating or delivering on these policy imperatives. Understanding the roles and experiences of frontline workers is crucial in understanding how frontline care can be made more 'person-centred'. The views of service users are also key in understanding how to promote independence.

'Frontline workers' is an umbrella term including all paid and voluntary workers who work directly with service users in the community. As the term implies, frontline workers are 'at the coal face' and have direct responsibility for the delivery of care. The qualities of frontline workers, their personal abilities and the training and support they are offered affect the care and support they provide and their ability to promote independence for the service user (Henwood and Waddington, 2002). With increasing numbers of frontline workers (Ford *et al.,* 1998), and a policy focus on community care, their roles are becoming more difficult to define (Cobban, 2004).

This review offers the opportunity to reflect explicitly on the role played by frontline workers in delivering a person-centred approach when working with older people, disabled people and people from minority ethnic communities. The review suggests ways to improve knowledge that could aid practice and better meet diverse needs of different community care groups.

The principal aim was to conduct a focused review of existing literature on the role of frontline workers within community care services. The review focused on frontline services for older people, disabled people and people from minority ethnic communities. There are a number of concerns raised within existing research relating to the delivery of care at the front line. These concerns relate both to the competency and qualities of individual frontline workers and the manner in which they are empowered and supported within their role. They also relate to systemic factors and management systems. These factors are explored within the review to illuminate the experiences of frontline workers caring for older people, disabled people and people from minority ethnic communities.

Methods

The literature review drew broadly on a systematic review approach. Details of what this involved can be found in Appendices 1 and 2.

We also engaged in a consultation process with service users and frontline workers. This involved facilitating four discussion groups and three focus groups.

Discussion groups

The aim of the discussion groups was to engage frontline workers and service users at an early stage of the study, and to ascertain how meaningful the themes we proposed to explore within the literature review were for both workers and users. The groups were composed of older people (nine participants); disabled people (eight participants); frontline workers in the social care field (eight participants); and frontline workers who were from and worked with service users from minority ethnic groups (four participants) working in the health care field.

Given the remit of the study, seven themes were explored:

- systemic management issues

- staff recruitment

- disempowerment and devaluing of frontline workers

- training/qualifications for frontline workers

- qualities of frontline workers

- working with families

- views on person-centred care

Focus groups

The focus groups aimed to explore the experiences of frontline workers and service users, and analyse how these findings related to the review of literature.

Nineteen participants were recruited through existing and new contacts with health, social and voluntary sector providers. Two groups were with frontline workers (one in Scotland and one in England) and one with service users (in Scotland). The focus group schedule is outlined in Appendix 3.

This study therefore draws together the review of the literature and the consultation exercise with frontline workers and service users. It does not evaluate existing services so cannot provide benchmarks for good person-centred care, nor does it identify examples of good practice. Chapter 5 does, however, suggest practical ways in which the findings of this study can be taken forward to better inform policy and practice.

2 PERSON-CENTRED CARE

This chapter has three aims: to assess the usage and meanings attached to the term 'person-centred', to present the evidence about what constitutes good-quality care/support and to highlight the importance of involving families in the care of service users.

Person-centred care

The term 'person-centred care' is mentioned frequently in the older people literature, particularly in dementia care, although the working definition of the concept is not always explicit. When person-centred care was first mooted in the dementia field it moved the focus from neurological impairment to the individual with dementia (Jacques and Innes, 1998). Ryan *et al.* (2004) noted that the new language within social policy now promotes person-centred care. However, what person-centred care means remains elusive.

Brooker (2004) highlights that, although the term is widely used by policy makers and practitioners in dementia care, there is a lack of consistency in how it is understood. Brooker (2004, p. 219) proposes that 'in person-centred care the relationships between all the people in the care environment should be nurtured'. Similarly, McCormack (2004) proposes that relationships, environmental conditions and individual values epitomise person-centred gerontological nursing.

Brooker (2004) proposes four elements that must be included to produce person-centred care:

- valuing people with dementia and those who care for them

- treating people as individuals

- looking at the world from the perspective of the person with dementia

- a positive social environment to enable the person with dementia to experience relative well-being.

McCormack's (2004) review on person-centred gerontological nursing concludes that there has been little research on what is meant by person-centred care and the impact person-centred care would have for users. Five approaches aiming to provide person-centred care are reviewed: Burford Nursing Development Unit approach; authentic consciousness; positive person work; the senses framework; and skilled companionship. McCormack (2004) concludes that person-centred nursing (or care) has four aspects:

- being in relation (social relationships)

- being in a social world (biography and relationships)

- being in place (environmental conditions)

- being with self (individual values).

Although McCormack's (2004) approach is more philosophical than Brooker's (2004), they have comparable features despite their different emphasis. McCormack (2004, p. 36) summarises the approach as 'the nurse as a facilitator of an individual's personhood' and 'the need for nurses to move beyond a focus on technical competence and requires nurses to engage in authentic humanistic caring practices that embrace all forms of knowing and acting, in order to promote choice and partnership in care decision-making'.

Further suggestions about what constitutes person-centred care within dementia care are: good communication (Bryan *et al.*, 2002); treating people as individuals (Moniz-Cook *et al.*, 2000; Cobban, 2004); and that, for person-centred care to occur, staff need person-centred management (Jacques and Innes, 1998; Ryan *et al.*, 2004).

Achieving person-centred care has received less attention. Two suggestions were identified in our review. First, Kharicha *et al.* (2004, p. 135) suggest that collaborative working and 'putting the needs of the patient at the centre of the care process' are crucial. However, they provide little evidence on the outcomes of collaborative working for users. This echoes McCormack's (2004) position about the lack of knowledge about the impact of person-centred care for service users.

Second, Moniz-Cook *et al.* (2000) argue that staff should receive training about 'person-centred care'. However, no clear definition is provided. The authors do suggest that knowing the life history of the individual and relating to residents as individuals are key aspects of quality care, which could be seen as constituents of 'person-centred care'.

Despite common parlance on 'person-centred care' in the older people and dementia literature, the reality of this was not reported by the older people who participated in the discussion group or focus groups for this study. Indeed, none of the service users participating in the discussion groups or focus group had heard of the term 'person-centred care'. When a definition was provided by the facilitator of the group, users felt that this did not describe the care they received.

Older people highlighted views on why they did not receive person-centred care, for example:

> ... physical problems of old age are not given the same attention as dementia.
>> (Field notes, older people discussion group)

Frontline workers working with people with dementia or older people (and disabled people) were familiar with the term. During focus groups, frontline workers defined person-centred care as:

> ... if you are being person centred then you will focus on what is important to them; it's not just their care needs it's also their social needs, their emotional needs, their family need. It is everything.
>> (Transcript, frontline worker focus group 2)

And:

> To treat someone as you would wish to be treated – someone like me to look after me.
>> (Transcript, frontline worker focus group 1)

Frontline workers also reported the surprise of service users when person-centred care was offered, suggesting that person-centred care was not necessarily a common occurrence for users:

> ... people have different reactions to person-centred care
> – some people are really surprised by being asked what
> their hopes and dreams are for the future – some people
> have never been asked such a question or been asked to
> think about things in that way.
> (Transcript, frontline worker focus group 1)

Person-centred planning (PCP)

While there was no direct reference to 'person-centred care'
within the literature reviewed for generic frontline workers or
disabled people, person centred planning (PCP) has been debated
as a way of working with people with learning difficulties. Magito-
McLaughlin *et al.* (2002) explore PCP as an alternative form of
support, while Parley (2001) looks at planning for care provision
under PCP in relation to quality outcomes. However, no major
decisions were made during the time of this study so he was
unable to assess the impact of this approach. Mansell and Beadle-
Brown (2004) review the evidence of PCP and point out that most
work discusses the process of PCP rather than outcomes for
users. Thus, there is no substantial evidence of its effectiveness
as a model of working.

Disabled participants did not feel that the services they received
were person centred in any way. This is summed up by the
comment:

> ... you take what you get, not what you want.
> (Field notes, disabled people discussion group)

Direct payments

Research on quality of care for disabled people has focused on
direct payments rather than person-centred care per se.

Participants in our disabled people discussion group had a vague knowledge of:

> ... 'self-payments' (direct payments) but they had no information about how it worked and how they could get this form of support.
>
> (Field notes, disabled user discussion group)

Direct payments successfully challenge rigid working practices and professional roles, and are perceived as opening up opportunities for social activity through flexibility and acknowledging users' needs for independent living (Kestenbaum, 1999). Carmichael and Brown (2002) suggest that direct payments improve the quality of life and confidence of service users, and increase the potential for disabled people to have more active lives, while Morris (1994) argues that they offer a way for the person with the disability to be at the centre of decision making about care/support services. In addition, Zarb and Nadash (1994) suggest that direct payments and associated payment schemes provide higher-quality support arrangements than direct service provision, give increased choice and control, and lead to greater levels of satisfaction with the support received.

This was the case for one focus group participant when beginning to use direct payments:

> I'm in control now ... I make the decisions, not some care company, I get what I need immediately ... not months down the line.
>
> (Transcript, user focus group)

Black and minority ethnic communities

Person-centred care for minority ethnic communities has been relatively unexplored. Suggestions for introducing a person-centred approach are: anti-discriminatory practices (Begum, 1995; Bowes and Dar, 2000b; Wilson, 2001); recognition and addressing of language barriers (Chambo and Ahmed, 2000); and the provision of specialist services (Gillam and Levenson, 1999; Bowes and Dar, 2000a; Menon *et al.*, 2001; Nemcek and Sabatier, 2003; Butt and O'Neill, 2004), which may employ black workers (Culley, 2000; Prevatt Goldstein, 2002). Such suggestions indicate a need to recognise cultural needs as a component of providing high-quality care.

Good-quality support/care

This discussion has shown that there are different emphases on 'person-centred care' for the user groups included in this review. The literature did highlight four factors that relate to 'good-quality support/care', all of which broadly adhere to the components of person-centred care above. Each of these are now considered.

Involving service users

Involving the service user in the planning and delivery of services can indicate a shift from a 'system' to a 'client' focus (Morris, 1994; Jones, 2001; Patmore, 2001; Roberts, 2002; Mansell and Beadle-Brown, 2004). Raynes *et al.* (2001) found that older people would like to meet regularly with providers, purchasers and elected members of care services in order to voice their concerns/ needs/opinions. Consulting with service users can lead to greater insight into the service they would prefer. For example, when consulted, home care service users felt that remaining at home allowed them to retain more control over their lives and that they preferred a 'low-key' approach to help (Cobban, 2004, p. 9).

The literature also stresses the importance of involving people with learning difficulties in decisions about care (Keywood *et al.*, 1999; Parley, 2001). However, service users who participated in this study did not always feel that services demonstrated a willingness to hear their views:

> ... social workers like to hear themselves speak [and not the service user].
> (Field notes, older people discussion group)

Even when frontline workers are keen to involve service users they identify limitations in practice:

> ... we have a young adult who is severely physically disabled, with a learning disability, we advocate for that person, hoping to win them round ... but there will be times when it will be challenging and we have to say that this is what this person wants ... advocating, negotiating.
> (Transcript, frontline worker focus group 2)

However, the benefits for users of being involved in the planning of their care were enthusiastically reported in this study, for example:

> ... makes me feel more human.
> (Transcript, service user focus group)

User views/needs

Vernon and Qureshi (2000) found that definitions of quality of care differ between service users and professionals. Service users' main concern is what the service does for them and how it is delivered (for example, if the behaviour of the carer is empowering). They also want control over the type of service received, particularly the timing of tasks and who provides the service. The importance of letting disabled children speak and treating them with respect has also been highlighted (Audit Commission, 2003).

Disabled people from minority ethnic communities face particular issues accessing services/support as a result of language, cultural and discriminatory barriers (Bignall and Butt, 2000; Vernon, 2002). Thus, there may be difficulties eliciting their views about their service needs.

Choice in services has been suggested as an indicator of quality care (Hardy *et al.*, 1999). However, the literature reveals a context where staff are concerned about difficulties with meeting need (Kestenbaum, 1999); with services being potentially budget rather than needs led (Priestley, 1998). This was an aspect of quality care seen as close to 'person-centred care':

> Services should be delivered with the person who gets the service being the one who identifies their needs.
> (Field notes, social care workforce discussion group)

The user focus group identified choice of services as a key feature of good-quality care/support:

> She can choose.
> (Transcript, service user focus group)

13

And:

> I can do things I've never done before [using direct
> payments to pay for help with activities of her choice].
> (Transcript, service user focus group)

Effective communication is seen as a key part of quality care. Language is argued to be more than just a communication tool (Chambo and Ahmed, 2000), with good communication also involving an understanding of factors such as culture, class and beliefs (Gillam and Levenson, 1999).

The literature also suggests that services focused on user views/needs may involve collaborative working between professionals (Wick *et al.,* 2003; Kharicha *et al.,* 2004; Ryan *et al.,* 2004) and can include direct consultation with service users (Gillam and Levenson, 1999; Raynes *et al.,* 2001). Both collaborative working and consultation with service users will require effective communication.

Continuity and reliability of care is an important aspect of care for older people (Patmore, 2001; Raynes *et al.,* 2001; SWRDU, 2002; Francis and Netten, 2004). The need to communicate changes is noted as particularly important:

> '… it is frightening to open your door to someone you
> don't know and whom you can't see. Couldn't someone
> phone me to say there's going to be a different person
> today?'
> (Raynes *et al.,* 2001, p. 2)

Promoting independence and autonomy

A common finding within the disability literature about good-quality care/support was the perception of good support services promoting independence and autonomy rather than control over the service user (Morris, 1994; Douglas *et al.*, 1998; Priestley, 1998; Davies *et al.*, 1999; JRF, 1999; Kestenbaum, 1999; Keywood *et al.*, 1999; Simons and Watson, 1999; Bignall and Butt, 2000; Vernon and Qureshi, 2000; Parley, 2001; Carmichael and Brown, 2002; Holborn and Vietze, 1999; Simon *et al.*, 2002; Stainton, 2002; Vernon, 2002; Audit Commission, 2003). Autonomy for service users has been suggested as a good indicator of high-quality care, as it is desirable, but difficult, to achieve (Davies *et al.*, 1999).

One young black disabled service user described the need for independence as:

'... having your own voice, you don't want anyone else to speak for you. If you're capable of speaking for yourself you should do'.

(Bignall and Butt, 2000)

This is not necessarily about living away from the family home, but having rights and some independence (Bignall and Butt, 2000).

The role of workers/services in promoting independent living for disabled people is also discussed in the literature (Morris, 1994; Douglas *et al.*, 1998, Priestley, 1998; Kestenbaum, 1999; Ungerson, 1999; Vernon and Qureshi, 2000), as is the divergence between independent living and community care policy (Morris, 1994; Priestley, 1998). Such literature highlights tensions in providing services that will achieve independence for service users.

Reliable and flexible services

The importance of flexibility, choice in services, control and individualised care to disabled people and older people has been robustly stated (Morris, 1994; Douglas *et al.*, 1998; Priestley, 1998; Hardy *et al.*, 1999; Kestenbaum, 1999; JRF, 1999; Simons and Watson, 1999; Vernon and Qureshi, 2000; Clark and Spafford, 2001; Patmore, 2001; Raynes *et al.*, 2001; Carmichael and Brown, 2002; Holborn and Vietze, 1999; Simon *et al.*, 2002; Stainton, 2002; SWRDU, 2002; Vernon, 2002; Hawthorne *et al.*, 2003; Francis and Netten, 2004), and is a key feature in perceptions of high-quality services.

Overcoming inflexibility in service provision is particularly important. Older people select direct payments, as they allow the flexibility to 'bank' hours for when needed (Clark and Spafford, 2001).

It has been argued that choice for users improves the quality of care (Hardy *et al.*, 1999). An example of the need to ensure choices are available throughout the assessment process can be found in the transition stage for disabled young people who do not experience an easy move from children's to adult services (Morris, 2002; Stalker, 2002).

Minority ethnic communities

The provision of services for minority ethnic groups exemplifies the challenge of ensuring flexibility and responsiveness. Service users reported better experiences of care from specialised services, but a focus on specialist services may stop mainstream services from improving (Bowes and Dar, 2000a, 2000b; Butt and O'Neil, 2004). Specialist voluntary services can provide valuable services and can help users with a range of problems such as accessing services, filling in forms and booking appointments (Chan and Cheung, 2004). However, voluntary specialised services have been found to be financially insecure (Butt and O'Neil, 2004) and are limited by both funding and a lack of qualified staff (Bowes and Dar, 2000a).

Frontline workers in this study supported the provision of specialist services:

> ... we have one worker who speaks a minority ethnic language and this is very important.
> (Transcript, frontline worker focus group 2)

And:

> ... specialist teams tend to take on minority ethnic service users.
> (Transcript, frontline worker focus group 2)

Suggestions to increase access to services for minority ethnic users are often simple. For example, in GP primary health care teams, more flexible appointment times would help minority ethnic populations with access (Hawthorne et al., 2003). Health and social care professionals report trying to take extra time and treat the service user as an individual, but say they have difficulties with inflexible working practices (Social Services Inspectorate, 1998; Gerrish, 2001).

Employing black workers has been suggested as a good way to provide services for black users but it is not clear if this is really the case (Blakemore, 1999; Culley, 2000; Prevatt Goldstein, 2002). Further, as minority ethnic workers are trained in the same systems as non-minority ethnic workers, their skill base may be similar. The problematic nature of this idea is also seen within geriatrics in the

National Health Service, where there are the highest numbers of minority ethnic workers, but where the services are least accessible for minority ethnic users (Culley, 2000).

Discussion group participants stressed that much of the success of their work came through personal experiences rather than formal training, which was often inadequate to address situations they encountered, while:

> ... the experiences they bring were unacknowledged by organisation.
>> (Field notes, minority ethnic health
>> frontline worker discussion group)

In addition, the need to work with a range of individuals, service users, family members and an array of frontline workers is essential:

> I need to be really diplomatic and work with them all.
>> (Transcript, frontline worker focus group 2)

Menon *et al.* (2001) recommend more frequent use of link workers and professional interpreters to improve access to services for minority ethnic communities. Gillam and Levenson (1999, p. 1215) suggest that link workers provide 'a cultural bridge between doctors and patients'. This has been found in the US where link workers (known as Community Health Workers) serve as a bridge between communities and professionals (Nemcek and Sabatier, 2003). In addition, Hawthorne *et al.* (2003) found that link workers improved relationships between health professional and minority ethnic service users. Link workers tend to be underused, however, as their role is not always understood.

The literature suggests that using link workers can improve the health of minority ethnic communities because of the strengthening of relationships between users and professionals leading to earlier identification of illness and earlier treatment (which can cut costs) and generally contributing to the reduction of health risks for minority ethnic communities (Khanchandani and Gillam, 1999; Nemcek and Sabatier, 2003).

Working effectively with families

If McCormack's (2004) four aspects of person-centred care are taken as a benchmark

- being in relation (social relationships)

- being in a social world (biography and relationships)

- being in place (environmental conditions)

- being with self (individual values),

families have a crucial role when undertaking person-centred care.

Listening to carer and user views

District nurses and GPs, who often have the first contact with carers, receive little training about carers' needs (Simon and Kendrick, 2001). Kestenbaum (1999) found that respite services were desirable to both carers and disabled people, but were not used in practice. There is also evidence (Keywood *et al.*, 1999) that carers can exert control over the services provided to people with learning difficulties, with service providers not listening to the views of people with learning difficulties but rather to the carer. In addition, parents and carers of disabled children often have to deal with several professionals but would prefer more co-ordination through, for example, a key worker (JRF, 1999).

Frontline workers in this study reinforced the value of working with families:

> ... to be in regular contact with the family is good for the family and for the service user.
>
> (Transcript, frontline worker focus group 1)

However, the potential for different accounts to emerge from families and users was reported as a challenge:

> If you go into one room with a carer and another room with the service user you get two completely different care plans!
>
> (Transcript, frontline worker focus group 2)

Relationships with carers and frontline workers

Hertzberg and Ekmann (2000) demonstrate that improving the relationship between staff and relatives can improve the care that older people in residential care receive. However, recognising and building relationships with families, from minority communities in particular, can be difficult, as this does not fit with western ideas and practices (Hawthorne *et al.*, 2003). Family and informal support can play a significant role in supporting young black disabled people (Bignall and Butt, 2000) and older people (Bond *et al.*, 1999), suggesting a need to ensure professionals and carers work together.

Frontline workers in this study highlight the tension in relationships between families and frontline workers:

> Family members were a source of information and a source of difficulties … 'interference' of family members … workers felt they were being monitored.
>
> (Field notes, social care worker discussion group)

And:

> … conflict in one family I work with where wife doesn't love him. We talk about it but I have to be careful … I have to stop at some point.
>
> (Transcript, frontline worker focus group 2)

Supporting service users and family relationships

Personal assistants (PAs) (using direct payments) can take pressure off family carers by both providing extra support and reducing tension within informal caring relationships (Ungerson, 1999), and can promote independence for both disabled people and their family members (Morris, 1994). Personal assistants can also mean disabled people have more choice about who comes to their home, and when and how the service is delivered (Carmichael and Brown, 2002). The literature also demonstrates that older people employing PAs can reduce dependence on family members and improve family relationships (Clark *et al.*, 2004).

Supporting the user may be the main goal of the frontline worker:

> … try to put the user first but family need to be involved.
>
> (Transcript, frontline worker focus group 2)

This suggests that, if workers are user orientated, they recognise the importance of the user/family relationship.

21

One service user also stressed her preference for her daughter not to be involved in her care, but for the frontline worker to be involved with her family:

> ... our daughter [name] helps now and again, but she has her own life and I just want her to come and talk, and I have [worker] and she is involved in the whole family.
> (Transcript, service user focus group).

Parents of disabled children identify information, advocacy, needs being met, emotional support and co-ordination of services as important (Middleton, 1998; JRF, 1999; Morris, 2002; Stalker, 2002; Audit Commission, 2003). Carers of older people benefit from support, advice, information and being involved in planning services (Lelliott *et al.*, 2003). However, research demonstrates that there can be a lack of empathy from staff for parents caring for disabled children, who have to fight for services and experience delays in appointments and services. Most commonly, parents felt that service providers gave poor information on services and lacked understanding of parents' experiences (Beresford, 1995). This may result in parents of disabled children exaggerating their child's needs in order to get ongoing rather than crisis-situation support (Middleton, 1998).

Achieving a balance of supporting the user and the carer may be difficult, as one male older service user reported:

> ... his sister had closer relationships with his home carers than he did.
> (Field notes, older people discussion group)

Further, the frontline worker needs to know when to withdraw to preserve the family relationship:

> I need to know when to pull away when not needed ...
> Workers can become possessive about clients.
>> (Transcript, frontline worker focus group 2)

Working with the whole family and understanding family dynamics was reported as usual in the minority ethnic frontline workers' discussion group. Cultural knowledge of the norms of family life was seen as useful, for example to understand that a family member may be the cause of the problem or that access to services may be controlled by a particular family member, thus preventing the person in need of care obtaining the support they require.

Conclusions

The term 'person-centred care' is not used consistently across the literature. However, McCormack's (2004) definition of being in relation, being in a social world, being in place and being with self can be linked to the three attributes of good-quality care, that is: the involvement of the service user; taking into account users' needs/views; and the provision of flexible and responsive services. Involving families in the care of people can be seen as an integral part of the provision of good-quality care if this involves listening to carers' and users' views; building relationships between frontline workers and carers; and supporting user and family relationships. This chapter demonstrates the complexity of 'person-centred care' and the range of tasks, duties and responsibilities that frontline workers must undertake should the care/support they provide be considered of high quality or 'person-centred'. Chapter 3 goes on to consider the personal skills and qualities needed from frontline workers to achieve this goal. However, even with the 'right' skill/quality/attribute mix, there are systemic challenges in providing person-centred/quality care (discussed in Chapter 4), which must also be addressed should person-centred care/quality care become a reality across client groups in the future.

3 PERCEPTIONS OF FRONTLINE WORK

The aim of this chapter is twofold. First, to present the evidence on the most important qualities of frontline workers in terms of their personal attributes, qualities and skills. Second, to explore the value attached to care work, both internally from service users, carers and management, and externally from other professions, the media and the general public.

Qualities of workers

Personal attributes

The personal attributes of frontline workers are often highlighted in research as influencing the relationship between worker and service user (SWRDU, 2002; Statham, 2004). Gender is a key attribute seen as facilitating the relationship between workers and service users (Lindesay and Skea, 1997; Jacques and Innes, 1998). Lindesay and Skea (1997) specifically note the significance of gender in the work of care assistants, with both male and female staff interacting more with male than female residents and female staff interacting more than male staff with all residents.

There is significant evidence that most frontline workers (Ford *et al.*, 1998; Thornley, 2000; UNISON, 2003; Foster, 2004) and many informal carers (Bond *et al.*, 1999; Harlow, 2004; Mansell and Beadle-Brown, 2004) are women. Indeed, women are said to make up 86 per cent of the social care workforce and constitute

78 per cent of field social workers (Harlow, 2004). There is also evidence to suggest that the majority of care workers are women approaching retirement age (SCWU, 2003). This highlights the relevance of both age and gender as key characteristics of those delivering care work, but tells us little about whether women, and specifically women approaching retirement age, are better equipped to offer the forms of care that are now required.

The consultation with frontline workers for this study suggests that more attention needs to be paid to gender in the delivery of care. There is increasing demand by service users to have a choice between male and female workers, in particular in the delivery of personal care.

For service users, there was a general awareness of the greater social acceptability of women offering caring services both to men and to women, relative to men doing so. Specifically, in relation to providing personal or intimate care:

> Some difficulties when a young man arrives as home help. Don't like to ask them to do particular tasks, for example ironing knickers – feel embarrassed asking men to do this.
>
> (Field notes, service user discussion group)

One man talked of having cared for his wife until she was taken into a nursing home and how the nursing home then took over his caring roles. He suggested his gender influenced his continuing caring role:

> I cared for my wife at home until she got too heavy, then we had carers come in to help with bathing her, and then later when she went into a nursing home they took over. I also have a friend whose husband is in a home. She

goes in every day to get him dressed and then at night to wash him and put him to bed. This makes me … I never got the opportunity, I would have liked to do more, but I was a man.

(Transcript, service user focus group)

These findings reinforce the notion of caring work as being 'women's work' (UNISON, 2003). Given this emphasis, respondents in this study suggest that the sexuality of men who work in caring jobs is often questioned. As one male care worker noted:

… [whether] I am gay is neither here nor there, but that is the immediate thought because I work in home care.

(Transcript, frontline worker focus group 2)

There was less evidence in both the literature and consultations of age being an important attribute of frontline workers. While age may be important in terms of who does perform caring roles, there is little evidence of age being recognised as important to being a good worker. The respondents in this study confirm this, with both frontline workers and service users recognising the need for both younger and older workers to bring different skills and experience. Attitude and motivation, both of which are discussed further below, were more important than age.

Bowes and Wilkinson (2003) point to both the gender and ethnicity of frontline workers being important in delivering dementia care services to minority ethnic groups. Minority ethnic frontline workers in this consultation confirm this, pointing out that it is women who perform the majority of formalised care work, and who are seen as more flexible and 'stretchable'. However, the lack of available male workers raises particular issues in meeting the needs of male service users within minority ethnic communities where gender segregation occurs.

Consultations with frontline workers emphasise that 'specialist' minority ethnic workers should meet the language and cultural needs of minority ethnic service users. This focus dominates over a view that all frontline workers could be suitably trained and culturally aware so as to offer culturally specific services to a diverse range of groups. This focus perhaps emerges from a lack of confidence or knowledge by generic workers, which may limit their capacity to work effectively with minority ethnic service users. But it is reinforced by a focus, within the literature and consultation, on promoting specialist services.

As Gillam and Levenson (1999) note, ethnicity is a key quality for workers working with minority ethnic groups, and can be promoted through the provision of specialist services. However, ethnicity is not everything; trust, class, culture and beliefs are important to providing appropriate care to minority ethnic groups. Most important are having a shared language and cultural understanding (Menon *et al.*, 2001; Chevannes, 2002; Vernon, 2002; Bowes and Wilkinson, 2003; Butt and O'Neill, 2004; Chan and Cheung, 2004).

Practical skills

In addition to personal attributes, practical skills are valued in the delivery of frontline health and care work. Skills such as moving and handling, personal care and domestic help are noted as particularly important (Ford *et al.*, 1998; Simons and Watson, 1999; Raynes *et al.*, 2001; Carmichael and Brown 2002; Finlayson *et al.*, 2002; Roberts, 2002; UNISON, 2003; Halliday and Asthana, 2004; Mansell and Beadle-Brown, 2004).

Simons and Watson (1999), in their review of day services for people with learning difficulties, note that there is an inverse relationship between the need for support by particular service users and the interaction of staff with this group. This disparity is thought to relate to the lack of skills of care staff in this setting. Butt and O'Neill (2004) similarly note that the cultural needs of minority ethnic older people are not being met by frontline workers, specifically relating to food and religious beliefs and practices. This suggests a lack of specific knowledge and skills by frontline workers, which limits their ability to fully undertake their role.

Training to meet the needs of specific client groups is therefore necessary to improve the skills base of frontline workers; in particular training that takes account of diversity in caring roles (Dalley and Denniss, 2001). Raynes et al. (2001) suggest that older people value carers who are trained to perform the necessary tasks for their role. Staff experience and skills are therefore identified as central to the attributes of frontline workers (Ford et al., 1998; Simons and Watson, 1999; Carmichael and Brown, 2002; Cockerill et al., 2002; Finlayson et al., 2002; Roberts, 2002; UNISON, 2003; Halliday and Asthana, 2004; Mansell and Beadle-Brown, 2004).

Personal qualities

A range of personal qualities are also noted as important to delivering frontline health and social care, including:

- patience, fortitude and compassion (Meek, 1998)

- warmth, reliability, honesty and empathy (Beresford, 2003)

- caring, kindness, understanding, gentleness, friendliness, helpfulness, willingness and thoughtfulness (Godfrey, 2000)

- showing 'respect, courtesy and maintaining confidentiality' (Cobban, 2004, p. 3)

- maintaining personal and professional values (Priestley, 1995; Ungerson, 1999; Parley, 2001; Wick *et al.*, 2003; Statham, 2004).

Godfrey (2000) found that both care staff and residents in nursing home settings cite personal qualities of staff as of central importance. Staff cite qualities such as 'communication, listening, patience, understanding, caring, humour, kindness and common sense' as important to their role, while residents cite 'patience, kindness, understanding and helpfulness' as central (Godfrey, 2000, p. 60). Further, both trained and untrained staff rate personal qualities above practical skills as important to performing their jobs (Godfrey, 2000).

Francis and Netten (2004) support this view, stating that respect, cheerfulness, friendliness, understanding and flexibility were key qualities of workers; with minority ethnic and white service users having the same needs in this respect. Further, a lack of flexibility is said to be the most problematic limitation in caring roles. A study by Meek (1998) on personal health care assistants found that users don't centrally value workers according to their skills and qualifications, but rather according to the personal qualities they bring to their work.

Frontline workers in this study talked about the difficulties they experienced in offering flexibility:

> ... at the end of the day you don't have the time to make a meal for someone.
>
> (Transcript, frontline worker focus group 2)

… we can't change what's in the diary.
>(Transcript, frontline worker focus group 2)

Some highlighted how they worked flexibly to offer better services, even if this is not what they are expected to do:

> Care workers are actually doing a lot more, they are changing the rota to do what the client wants done. We have days when we go to the shop, take them to the hairdresser.
>(Transcript, frontline worker focus group 2)

> I have a gentleman that can't go out so I go and get him a paper … I have another gentleman who likes cooked chicken. It's just things that are not down on your list.
>(Transcript, frontline worker focus group 2)

Service users similarly value flexibility. Help with specific household chores, running errands or simply having a cup of tea together were seen as important to the service received. However, both service users and frontline workers recognise the limits of this in practice with increasing constraints on services, as one service user notes:

> … two weeks ago there was a review. The team leader said they would be cutting [husband's] care hours, but he can't get in and out of the chair! … So now my personal carer helps both him and me. He was refused extra care for so long, now he has been given half an hour for a shower each night. But it's ridiculous, that's not enough time to give a person in a wheelchair a shower – in half an hour!
>(Transcript, service user focus group)

The concern here is the rigid time allocations offered for specific tasks and how this impacts on both service users and frontline workers.

While many clients would like company, frontline workers are not always offering their time for this, with some frontline workers performing only the tasks they are allocated to do. If their tasks take less than the allocated time there is a view from some frontline workers that they should not stay to offer company. In short, some staff are being more rigid in following the rules than others; staff have different styles of working, different priorities for their time and different views on how to deal with requests for additional support.

Caring as a relationship

Underpinning this discussion is a more fundamental issue about how the qualities of workers help frame the relationship between service users, their families and frontline workers.

Several research reports cite a central motivation of health and care workers is to gain job satisfaction directly from performing their caring roles (Penna *et al.*, 1995; Cockerill *et al.*, 2002; Finlayson, 2002; Roberts, 2002). Public sector workers choose this work, as it offers the opportunity to make a positive difference to the lives of service users and local communities (Audit Commission, 2002), while care workers cite a commitment to caring as well as the flexibility associated with the work as central motivations for performing this work (Ford *et al.*, 1998). While a range of personal attributes, skills and qualities of workers are identified as central to performing caring roles, it is the centrality of the motivation to care that is found to drive health and social care workers to perform their roles:

> I am very caring, the client is the sole concern for me.
>> (Transcript, frontline worker focus group 1)

> I love my work ... We care!
>> (Transcript, frontline worker focus group 2)

Staff morale is linked, not only to pay, working environment, staffing levels and workload, but also to the pressure of work, feeling valued and supported, and gaining satisfaction from their work (Finlayson, 2002). Clearly, then, what motivates staff is more complex than merely the satisfaction of offering care and support, but how this fits alongside a range of measures of satisfaction. Nonetheless, frontline workers identify job satisfaction as centrally related to their contact with service users and the perceived progress that is being made with them (Penna *et al.*, 1995).

The relationship with the service user is therefore central to frontline caring roles (Douglas *et al.*, 1998; Ungerson, 1999; Vernon and Qureshi, 2000; Henwood, 2001). Achieving this comes through giving service users more control over who it is that provides care, specifically through the use of personal assistants (Morris, 1994; Zarb and Nadash, 1994; Ungerson, 1999), through frontline workers playing a role in promoting autonomy for older people (Davies *et al.*, 1999) and through a commitment to joint working as a means of putting the person at the centre of the care process (Kharicha *et al.*, 2004).

Consultations with frontline workers and older service users similarly note the importance of positive relationships between worker and service user:

> ... we are with these people for years, we become part of the family, we think about them.
>> (Transcript, frontline worker focus group 1)

> I have a man that I go to who I spend time cleaning up and getting dressed. By the time I leave he is all clean and smart. I feel really good about that, and he does too. I enjoy that feeling of doing that, of making him feel better.
> (Transcript, frontline worker focus group 2)

Older service users comment specifically on the value of continuity with the same worker over time. Several are concerned both about occasions when their usual carer is absent (due to illness or holidays) and what will happen when their carer moves on to another job or retirement. Building new relationships and establishing trust are therefore central to caring roles. Thus, frontline workers are seen in relation to their interpersonal skills and the long-term bond that is built with those they work with.

As discussed in Chapter 2, it is important to put the person first in caring situations. Working with families is also an essential element of the job, with family members offering an important source of information about service users:

> Families must be involved. When my wife lost her speech, I was the only one who knew her likes and dislikes. For example, she hated being called Janet. I had to pass that information on to social workers and carers.
> (Transcript, service user focus group)

Family and neighbours often offer informal care alongside or in place of more formal caring roles performed by frontline health and social care professionals (Bond *et al.*, 1999; Lelliott *et al.*, 2003).

However, difficulties were noted about finding time to support family members in their caring roles:

> Finding time to spend with carers is really difficult on top of seeing clients and doing paperwork. I've had carers crying … We need to support them … I don't have time in a 15-minute slot to do that.
>
> (Transcript, frontline worker focus group 2)

This highlights the need for frontline care staff to be equipped with a range of skills that will allow them to manage relationships with family members as well as with service users. It also highlights the tensions that can arise between meeting the needs of service users and family members when these may not always be in alignment.

Value of care work

As well as the personal qualities of frontline workers, there is extensive debate on the value attributed to care work by others; it is to this issue that attention now turns.

Professional value

Frontline workers recognise their work as valuable and worthwhile, with satisfaction gained from performing their caring roles. However, morale of workers is affected by the value placed on their roles by both their own managers and other professionals. Lack of qualifications was particularly noted as affecting the perceived value of care assistants; while different qualification levels between different workers is suggested as potentially causing tension and devaluing less qualified staff within the profession (Jacques and Innes, 1998; Perry *et al.*, 2003).

Similarly, home care has traditionally been afforded a low status in the workplace (Workman, 1996; Cobban, 2004). Care assistants working in care homes cite a lack of training as leading to a poor skills base, low professional status and poor self-esteem (Dalley and Denniss, 2001). The result is a disparity in value associated with some frontline care roles relative to others.

One explanation for this is that home care workers are seen by management as a cheaper option than more qualified staff (Aronson and Neysmith, 1996). The time required to perform their tasks and the emotional work they perform is both overlooked and undervalued. Home care workers often do more than their formal tasks, and thus ignore formal working regulations (SWRDU, 2002). Management is seen as complicit in this by praising staff for doing extra (unpaid) work (Aronson and Neysmith, 1996), while not valuing them professionally as workers with a particular set of skills.

Cobban (2004), and respondents in this study, note the lack of contact between frontline and management staff in their day-to-day work, and a lack of formal supervision/support from management. This does not mean that staff do not get support when required, but suggests a lack of recognition of the interpersonal and potentially challenging roles performed by frontline staff and the possibility of needing formal support mechanisms to be in place.

Minority ethnic frontline workers involved in this study talked of their line managers as potentially providing useful support and encouragement, but that in practice this is more problematic. Too much emphasis has been placed on promoting advocacy and interpreting both by management and other professionals, with little or no acknowledgement of the other skills workers have to offer. Alongside this, suggestions for practice offered by frontline workers are often ignored; an example of this came when management refused to use the term 'refugee' despite it being the most appropriate term and one used by service users and frontline workers. The term was later accepted, but not as a result of the influence of frontline staff. Minority ethnic frontline workers felt their expertise was being drawn on but rarely acknowledged.

Other professionals are also identified as undervaluing particular forms of frontline work. As one participant notes:

> I find nursing staff, 'look down' is too strong, but they give out instructions to a home carer as if they were more knowledgeable about what the home carers do ... I've had complaints [from clients] because they feel degraded by nurses ... I am not saying all nurses, as some are very nice people, but I am aware perhaps of the way things are going now. It used to be a lot of what we are doing was done by nurses, personal care wise.
>
> (Transcript, frontline worker focus group 2)

Another respondent illustrates how this division between professional groups has manifested itself in terms of nurses' attitudes to home care staff:

> We had a situation recently where a home care worker arrived at a client's home and there was a nurse there who had given the client an enema. The nurse said she had to go to her next job and that the home care worker would have to stay to help the client go to the toilet. But the problem is that she didn't have time to do that, she only had a 15-minute slot with this client ... We are not able to give 100 per cent with that sort of thing going on.
>
> (Transcript, frontline worker focus group 2)

One respondent who was previously a nurse recognises this division:

> I'm a nurse and there is a sense of that ... I used to think that we are a profession and we specialise.
>
> (Transcript, frontline worker focus group 2)

This highlights a particular concern from home care workers about their value relative to other caring professionals. Domiciliary care workers also see their work as being undervalued relative to registered nurses (UNISON, 2003). This highlights significant differences between professional groups, with qualifications seen as of higher value than the qualities and attributes offered by home care and domiciliary care workers.

Social value

Government policy arguably reinforces this view of some professional groupings as having higher value than others; with much more policy attention currently given to addressing recruitment and retention issues in nursing than to the position of home care workers (see Finlayson, 2002; Finlayson *et al.*, 2002; King's Fund, 2004). Our consultations confirms this:

> ... they need to put more value on our services, we hear about nurses, but what about us?
>   (Transcript, frontline worker focus group 2)

Other participants point to the lower status afforded to home care workers relative to health visitors, social workers, etc., with service users expecting home care workers to wait if they arrived when another professional was in attendance, stating that 'it's only the home help'. This implies that their workload and role are less valued than other health and social care professionals.

While policy frameworks may acknowledge the role of frontline workers, there is a sense that the public does not understand how work patterns and demands have shifted in recent years, with responsibilities with regard to delivering services now much greater (UNISON, 2003). Public attitudes to frontline health and social care work are therefore potentially uninformed in terms of the type of work performed and the issues frontline workers face in their caring roles. For example, Penna *et al.* (1995) point to the regularity of experiences of verbal and physical abuse at work faced by residential care staff.

Consultations with some generic frontline workers highlight a lack of recognition by service users and their families of the work undertaken. Little attention is given to the skills possessed and there is a view from some that service users and their families want a lot from the service while not recognising the work involved. However, this view is not shared by all:

> ... we get letters all the time, gifts and cards.

> ... we are devalued by society, but our job satisfaction comes from the users.

> ... they tell you if they're happy.

> ... and if they aren't.
>   (Transcript, frontline workers focus group 1)

Added to this is the value attributed to the work from family and friends:

> ... my friends and family think I have the best job in the world but publicly, externally, it is negative. There is nothing good said about my job.
>   (Transcript, frontline worker focus group 1)

... the people I know see it as good work, I get positive feedback and am treated with a lot of respect.
>
> (Transcript, frontline worker focus group 2)

A lack of understanding by the public of the work involved is offered as a partial explanation for the low value attributed to this work:

... people aren't really aware of us until they need the service ... but people don't hold it in high regard.
>
> (Transcript, frontline worker focus group 2)

Within minority ethnic communities there is a view that some forms of health and social care work are valued less than others for both men and women. While there are cultural differences between groups, minority ethnic respondents noted that being a doctor is thought to be acceptable, but not a nurse or a social worker:

From the ethnic minority scene it is not valued ... a waste of brains to go into social work ... it is not valued work.
>
> (Transcript, frontline worker focus group 2)

This suggests a need to focus on valuing frontline workers alongside service users (Reed et al., 2003; Brooker, 2004):

... you have to think about the staff in a person-centred way too.
>
> (Transcript, frontline worker focus group 2)

As Ryan *et al.* (2004) state, frontline workers need to be valued from a range of sources: by service users and carers; by their organisation; and by wider society.

One aspect of frontline work that potentially has more positive value is specialist services. There is evidence that specialist physical disability social workers (Kestenbaum, 1999) and key workers supporting families with disabled children (Mukherjee *et al.*, 1999) may be more valued than general social workers. As noted in Chapter 2, personal assistants support family carers (Witcher *et al.*, 2000) both by providing services and by reducing tension within informal caring relationships (Ungerson, 1999). Recent evidence of personal assistance for older people similarly suggests a reduction in dependence on family members and improved family relationships as potential gains (Clark *et al.*, 2004). One study found that a lack of specialist frontline workers was limiting the usefulness of some services for people with learning difficulties (Cambridge and McCarthy, 2001). In short, specialist or more individualistic services that concentrate on holistic or expert approaches to delivering support offer the most positive models of working, and are therefore most valued both by service users and family members.

Conclusions

This chapter has reviewed the qualities of frontline workers and the value attached to frontline health and social care work by others. What has emerged is a picture where frontline workers highlight their personal commitment to health and social care work, and to a lesser extent the importance of frontline workers having a set of personal attributes relating to gender, ethnicity and skills that equip them to perform this role. Given the central importance of personal qualities over professional training, it is interesting to note that there is a different value placed on workers depending on their professional status.

In terms of the value associated with frontline work, it seems that lack of knowledge of the tasks performed by frontline workers stands as the greatest barrier to a positive image of this role. Further, it is suggested that there is a higher status accorded to specialist provision than to generic workers, which is perhaps unsurprising given that specialist workers often have a level of expertise or are able to be flexible in the provision of services in a way that generic workers frequently do not have the time or resources to accommodate.

The general messages that emerge are that more acknowledgement needs to be given to the emotional labour employed in this work, to the centrality of a commitment to caring and to the personal qualities that are so valued by service users and family carers. Further, the value attributed to frontline health and social care work by managers, other professionals, the public and Government suggests too much attention to the professional status of workers, and not enough to the qualities that frontline health and social care workers both deliver and offer. Further, the changing role of home care workers means they are far more likely to be asked to perform personal care tasks carried out traditionally by health visitors. In light of this, more attention needs to be given to the skills that this group of workers do possess and the importance of these to both frontline workers and service users.

4 SYSTEMIC AND ORGANISATIONAL ISSUES FOR FRONTLINE WORKERS

This chapter discusses organisational and systemic issues that frame and influence the experiences of frontline workers and service users. It explores broad systemic issues currently impacting on the role of frontline workers; the management of frontline workers; training for frontline workers; and the recruitment of frontline workers.

Systemic issues

The main systemic issues highlighted in the literature relate to changes in commissioning and budgeting systems, which have led to decreasing resources and increasing bureaucracy for frontline workers (Rummery and Glendinning, 2000; Jones, 2001; Foster, 2004; Harlow, 2004). ADSW (2004) highlights systemic issues such as the impact of the modernisation agenda and increasing emphasis on a performance culture – issues that are echoed by Harrison and Smith (2003). Ellis *et al.* (1999) highlight increasing tension in the social worker's role between administrative structures and professional approaches to service users. Systemic constraints limit the potential for user-led services (Kersten *et al.*, 2000). Harlow (2004) similarly points to the increased managerial responsibility that now goes with social work as a result of a greater focus on costs of services and new skills in purchasing and contracting. This managerial refiguration of social work means a transformation of this work. Increasing bureaucracy was noted by the frontline workers and service users in this study as a negative aspect of providing care:

> Staff rearrangements are the problem, constantly being restructured and this means no one really knows what is going on ... too much bureaucracy.
>
> (Transcript, service user focus group)

Policy changes have led to changes in the role of frontline workers. For example, home helps are 'now increasingly providing complex and intimate personal care packages and targeting these newer services towards those with the greatest need' (Cobban, 2004, p. 50). Penna et al. (1995) acknowledge increased work pressure for residential care workers who perceive service users as having greater needs. The result is that domiciliary care workers see a change in the nature of their work (UNISON, 2003). Cooking, cleaning and shopping are no longer central and staff are increasingly providing care associated with nursing. Frontline workers in this study reinforce this view:

> There are [now] different criteria for what kinds of clients they help. Some clients are now missing out on care. This is due to government standards.
>
> (Transcript, frontline worker focus group 1)

Restrictive budgets and commissioning structures can limit resources and flexibility, affecting the amount of time frontline workers have to spend with service users and the range and individuality of the services they provide (Morris, 1994; Davis et al., 1998; Priestley, 1998; Hardy et al., 1999; Mukherjee et al., 1999; Rummery and Glendinning, 2000; Jones, 2001; Simon et *al.*, 2002, SWRDU, 2002; Cobban, 2004; Francis and Netten, 2004; Halliday and Asthana, 2004). Commissioning restrictions caused by local authorities contracting out care mean time slots may be set, which denies user choice and flexibility (SWRDU, 2002; Cobban, 2004). Restrictive commissioning often means home care workers have insufficient time and may turn up late leading to unreliability for service users (Francis and Netten, 2004). Lack of time is commonly reported by home care workers (Cobban, 2004). The frontline workers consulted here emphasised time as a limited resource and one that restricted their ability to provide good care for service users. They agreed that time limits meant they were not able to chat and provide company for the service users. Older service users commented that frontline workers seldom had time to stay and chat. Some felt these restrictions were greater in larger organisations, such as local authorities, while independent or voluntary organisations offered greater flexibility:

> ... it is a basic value ... if you don't have the resources, it's not a case of having two clients to do in an afternoon, you will have six clients and the same amount of resources ... the time isn't available. When I started I had two hours per client, I could spend time with the client, have some rapport with the client, get to know them. Now I am lucky ... I am sure you would agree that home carers say they are lucky if they get 30 minutes in the morning, 30 minutes at lunchtime and at night-time.
> (Transcript, frontline worker focus group 2)

Other restraints reported by home care workers relate to what they are 'allowed' to do (SWRDU, 2002; Cobban, 2004). Morris (1994) argues that statutory providers are inflexible in the way they deliver services. This inflexibility includes: lack of choice for

45

service users about how support is provided, lack of opportunities to use support to participate in activities outside home, too much focus on caring and cleanliness rather than independence and a reduction in services (Morris, 1994). There is a general tendency to fit the client to the service rather than the service to the client, thus creating dependence on services at the convenience of provider rather than service user. Morris (1994) further argues that statutory provision similar to residential provision creates incarceration in the home rather than in an institution. This is echoed by a frontline worker consulted in this project:

> I think we are going back to more institutional ... they are closing them down, but they are keeping institutionalisation out in the community.
> (Transcript, frontline worker focus group 2)

Lack of resources limits real choice for users (Hardy et al., 1999). Rummery and Glendinning (2000) note that frontline practitioners and managers may limit access to resources through limiting the number of applicants accessing a full community care assessment. This suggests that many frontline services are budget led rather than needs led (Priestley, 1998). The more responsibility for working within tight resource restrictions is devolved to frontline staff, the greater the risk is that professional judgements will be subject to managerial pressures to stay within budget (Rummery and Glendinning, 2000). Frontline workers and service users in this study were in agreement that a lack of resources for frontline care services was severely limiting their efficacy.

Penna et al. (1995) highlight the perception that, in order to save money, local authorities are freezing posts, shifting to part-time contracts and inferior conditions of service, reorganising shift systems and relying increasingly on casual staff. They also note that staff shortages result in increased workloads, demoralisation and a feeling of being constantly under pressure. This in turn has a negative effect on service users. Service users value consistency in the service they receive (Patmore, 2001), but report that resource constraints limit staff cover for sickness and absence, leading to inconsistent and unsatisfactory service provision:

> Main issue is the number and availability of staff – services always seem to be short staffed.
> (Field notes, older people discussion group)

Low rates of pay, poor working conditions and failure of human resources strategies are bad for morale, as there is a feeling that employers are not acknowledging the demands of frontline work and the value of frontline workers' contributions (UNISON, 2003). Social workers are identified as experiencing more stresses in their job resulting from lack of consultation on changes in service, more regulated and mundane contact with clients, more administration and more pressure to quantify their work (Jones, 2001). As the response to the following question illustrates:

> So would you say the way your services are structured is a barrier to person-centred care?
>
> Several reply 'Yes!'
> (Transcript, frontline worker focus group 2)

Frontline workers do, however, try to provide good care even when the system is against them (SWRDU, 2002; Wick et al.,

2003). Frontline workers aspire to good teamworking. In nursing homes, teams are found to have shared goals and an understanding of each other's contributions (Wick *et al.*, 2003). The frontline workers in this study did try to work around the system. Service users spoke of different types of workers, some willing to bend rules and others not willing:

> The home carers are person centred because we do do extras, we do do things that we are not supposed to do. And we do meet the clients' needs, we will go to the shops ... it is these little things that make the difference.
> (Transcript, focus group 2)

> Staff may undertake 'underground' work to offer a fuller service to a user overruling the will of management.
> (Field notes, minority ethnic health frontline worker discussion group)

Management

The management of frontline workers is also affected by the issues discussed above. Statham (2004) argues that models of management currently used within social work are more concerned with command and control; they promote the belief that, within social work practice, structures are more important than relationships with service users. Similarly, Foster (2004) notes that social work practices are undervalued while structures, procedures and management are overemphasised. A lack of management and social support is one of a range of difficulties social workers face (Jones, 2001). At one of the focus groups in this study frontline workers and their management were present.

It was clear from the discussions that there was tension based on a lack of understanding of each other's roles. Minority ethnic frontline workers also reported this tension and felt their managers did not understand or value their work, with managers seeming to be more focused on quantifiable outputs. Boehm and Staples (2002) suggest that social care managers are under increasing pressure to stick to budgets.

The quality of management in health and social care is often found to be poor. Ford *et al.*'s (1998) study reports poor management and poor supervisory practices, while Halliday and Asthana (2004) report that link workers suggest a lack of support from their managers in their role. Care home managers often have a lot of experience of care but little or no formal training on management skills (Johnson *et al.*, 1999). Hierarchical management systems in nursing homes may hinder teamworking and weak, poor managers exacerbate these problems, creating factions among staff and fostering distrust (Wick *et al.*, 2003). One manager highlights the difficulties of management:

> … as a manager I don't get much of the 'nice stuff'. I get the complaints.
> (Transcript, frontline worker focus group 1)

Both frontline workers and service users consulted within this study stated that, in general, there was a lack of support from managers for frontline workers. Huge differences were found between individual experiences about levels of support from management:

> … we have a very good system … as a rule we meet every six weeks for formal supervision.

49

... there is not enough management.

I meet my manager once a week ... they are terrific ...
previous one was 'alright' that is the best I could say.
(Transcript, frontline worker focus group 2)

Good management can improve the experience of frontline workers and the quality of care they deliver. Penna *et al.*'s (1995) study of residential care workers found that good teamwork and supportive management were key factors in mediating workplace stress. The qualities cited as supportive in managers were approachability, willingness to listen and ability to respond in a way not perceived as undermining to staff.

A lack of knowledge among managers may limit the range of services available to service users. Direct payments are reported as a positive option by older people but they require support services for the financial and recruitment aspects of direct payments (Clark and Spafford, 2001; Clark *et al.*, 2004). Direct payments are still to become the norm for older people, and lack of knowledge and negative attitudes towards them among care managers limit access for older people (Clark and Spafford, 2001).

The systemic and management issues discussed above are exacerbated for minority ethnic groups. The cultural characteristics of these groups may make some systems harder to access and changes to systems more confusing (Hawthorne *et al.*, 2003). Frontline health staff felt frustrated, angry and helpless due to communication and cultural barriers, and due to systemic issues that do not fit with the expectations or behaviour of minority ethnic service users (Hawthorne *et al.*, 2003).

Minority ethnic service users and frontline workers are further disadvantaged by a lack of managers from minority ethnic communities (Hunter, 2003). A survey conducted by Hunter (2003) found a lack of minority ethnic workers at high levels within social services. Out of 187 social work directors only one was from a minority ethnic community. The survey further found that managers from minority ethnic communities are more qualified than white managers at the same level, suggesting discrimination within recruiting systems (Hunter, 2003).

Training

Frontline workers have a range of training experiences but few receive sufficient appropriate and effective training. Lack of resources limits access to training for frontline workers (Morris, 1994; Dalley and Denniss, 2001; Cobban, 2004; Francis and Netten, 2004). Practical difficulties, such as cost, availability and quality of courses, contributed to difficulties in providing training for care assistants (Dalley and Denniss, 2001). There are inequalities in the training offered to different types of workers in different organisations (Ford *et al.*, 1998; Pickard *et al.*, 2003; Dalley and Denniss, 2001):

> I had no training just a quick induction. Going on my first job was terrifying, I didn't know what to do.

> ... different organisations have different training. There is no standard approach and I wonder if we should have one?
> (Transcript, frontline worker focus group 1)

For home care workers, lack of resources means that training on practical issues such as moving and handling gets priority while resource restraints limit access to training on other topics (Cobban, 2004). Frontline staff consulted here had mixed experiences of

51

training. Most found that generic, basic courses such as lifting and handling were common while more specialised and more useful training courses were difficult to access:

> ... training isn't any good ... we do a lot of physical training ... hoisting, lifting and carrying, personal care ... we are not taught communication skills, how to enhance communication.
>
> (Transcript, frontline worker focus group 2)

There are questions about the suitability and efficacy of training (Ford *et al.*, 1998; Meek, 1998; Davies *et al.*, 1999; Godfrey, 2000; Stalker, 2002; Cobban, 2004). Training has not kept up with changing needs of users and expectations of workers. The literature raises specific training needs for staff working with disabled people – for example, the need for more staff to get disability equality training (Stalker, 2002) and training about being a key worker (Halliday and Asthana, 2004). A disability worker consulted during this project noted that the increasing use of direct payments has led to service users being responsible for the training of their personal assistants. This type of training is seen as appropriate, allowing frontline workers to effectively meet the needs of their service users. It is important that funding for personal assistants takes account of training costs (Morris, 1994). One report found that service users wish access to training to enable them to be involved in their own care planning (JRF, 1995).

Staff have reported the benefits of training as providing 'confidence, knowledge and experience' (Godfrey, 2000, p. 60). In this study frontline workers emphasised the importance of training:

… individual support is crucial for staff. Staff need to have time to review work and build up positive relationships with carers. Training is very important.
(Transcript, frontline worker focus group 1)

Lack of training for care assistants in care homes has led to an associated poor self-image and low status (Dalley and Denniss, 2001). The attainment of qualifications affects the perceived value placed on care assistants and other staff, and may cause tension and lead to the devaluing of less qualified staff (Jacques and Innes, 1998). In addition, those who are lowest paid and have lowest status have the fewest opportunities for training (SCWU, 2003). This is compounded by a lack of recognition of the skills frontline workers gain through experience (Moniz-Cook et al., 1997).

Training is seen by many care home managers as beneficial to the quality of care residents receive (Dalley and Denniss, 2001). However, some managers believe training leads to an increase in staff turnover (Dalley and Denniss, 2001), suggesting a complex relationship between training and quality of care (Davies et al., 1999; Dalley and Denniss, 2001). Studies on specific training report benefits – for example, better knowledge of home care workers about dementia improves the care they deliver (Cobban, 2004). Moniz-Cook et al. (2000) found that training in person-centred care may change the perception of challenging behaviour, while Davies et al. (1999) found a positive relationship between the level of education of frontline staff in care homes and resident autonomy. Specific training on working with people with communication problems was found to significantly benefit frontline staff, as it challenged staff attitudes to communication and increased knowledge in this area (Bryan et al., 2002).

Research suggests that a training focus on both personal skills and practical skills is useful to develop 'good' care workers

(Godfrey, 2000). Godfrey (2000) found that residents liked staff more the longer they were in the job, regardless of the amount of training. Another study found that older people value carers who are trained in appropriate tasks and who are trained to listen (Raynes *et al.*, 2001). Training has been found to be of particular importance when working with minority ethnic service users (Bowes and Dar, 2000b; Menon *et al.*, 2001; Chevannes, 2002). Training on minority ethnic issues is needed for both minority ethnic and non-minority ethnic frontline staff in both health and social care (Social Services Inspectorate, 1998; Menon *et al.*, 2001; Hawthorne *et al.*, 2003). Specific training is needed to learn how to work with and use interpreters (Gerrish, 2001). The frontline workers consulted for this study support this:

> … training on ethnic minority issues … is lapse. My own area has a large Muslim population but there is no education on what I could or could not do when I first arrived.
> (Transcript, frontline worker focus group 2)

> … minority ethnic and black older people do come into residential care but their needs are different – skin and hair care – so need specialist training and input.
> (Transcript, frontline worker focus group 1)

There is some evidence that minority ethnic training for non-minority ethnic staff can have negative effects, as they are afraid of causing offence or acting inappropriately (Bowes and Dar, 2000b). However, some training on minority ethnic issues was found to increase awareness of racial stereotyping by white workers and improve their understanding of local resources (Chevannes, 2002). Training was found to change the thinking and increase the confidence of frontline workers, some of whom were concerned about being seen as racist (Chevannes, 2002). However, the majority of workers found training difficult to put into practice because of their workplace practices (Chevannes, 2002).

Recruitment

There is a strong indication that recruitment and retention are problems for employers of frontline workers (Audit Commission, 2002; McFarlane and McLean, 2003; SCWU, 2003; UNISON, 2003; ADSW, 2004; Harlow, 2004; King's Fund, 2004). UNISON (2003) reports that social work rates of pay are declining relative to other public sector workers, leading to an absolute shortage of social workers willing to join the workforce. Harlow (2004) states that women leave social work as a result of stress, workload, changes in the nature of the job, low pay, low status, loss of professional autonomy and poor promotion prospects. There has also been a growing problem with staff recruitment with a reduction in applications to social work courses (Harlow, 2004). Harlow (2004) further argues that women now have other career options and more individual freedom so are no longer choosing social work as a career option to the same degree. An Audit Commission (2002) report found that 'push' factors are encouraging people to leave the public sector. These include: bureaucracy; lack of autonomy; insufficient resources; feeling undervalued by managers; pay that is not felt fair compared with others doing similar work; and a change agenda that can feel imposed and irrelevant. Problems of recruitment in nursing are leading to more use of agency nurses and non-UK citizens to fill gaps (Buchan et al., 2004), and recruitment and retention issues are compounded by staff absences and inability to cover workload (Jones, 2000, 2001). Frontline workers consulted here did not highlight recruitment and retention as problems, reporting little staff turnover within their organisations:

> ... not at mine!

> ... not high in day care, not in my last organisation. This is a lot to do with the support that is given in this job ... if people feel they have training, feel valued they will stay.
> (Transcript, frontline worker focus group 1)

This inconsistency may be due to the limited scope of this study and may also reflect that recruitment and retention are not important issues for frontline workers. The frontline workers did, however, highlight issues about long-term absence and problems replacing experienced staff. One stated that good pay meant that staff did not leave their jobs but would go on long-term absence, putting pressure on other staff. Frontline workers and service users both spoke of a lack of consistency among home care staff and problems with replacing experienced staff.

There is a need to recruit more workers from minority ethnic communities (Social Services Inspectorate, 1998; Hunter, 2003). However, there are problems both with recruitment and with the subsequent development of minority ethnic workers. Culley (2000) explored equal opportunities for nurses in the UK and found minority ethnic nurses face racism from service users and colleagues. Promotion is often slower for minority ethnic nurses and there is some evidence that they are discriminated against in the recruitment process (Culley, 2000). Minority ethnic workers are often in junior posts and employed for cultural skills while their own professional development is not seen as important (Bowes and Dar, 2000b). Prevatt Goldstein (2002) finds that minority ethnic workers are exploited for their cultural skills, but the additional work they do is seldom acknowledged. The minority ethnic frontline workers in this study echoed this, reporting that managers often require their expertise but seldom give recognition for this. They also stressed the difficulties in finding and recruiting new minority ethnic frontline staff:

> ... recruitment an issue too, not enough black and bilingual workers for older people ... But will be more older Chinese people soon, need to prepare staff now, recruit people now, encourage people to get into the frontline workers, especially social work.
>
> (Transcript, service user focus group)

Conclusions

Systemic and organisational factors appear to pose barriers to the provision of person-centred care and the promotion of independence by frontline workers. Increasing bureaucracy, tighter budgets and restrictive commissioning of services all limit the ability of frontline workers to provide quality care to service users. The impact of these factors on limiting time available for care and support was the main issue emphasised by frontline workers and service users consulted within this study. These limitations cause additional stress for frontline workers already working in stressful conditions.

Poor and inconsistent management of frontline workers further hinders their ability to provide quality care. Social and health care managers are increasingly under pressure to stay within given budgets and this causes conflict with the roles of frontline workers. It seems that immediate line managers may be supportive while higher-level managers place less value on the work done by frontline workers. There is also a mixed picture of the training received by frontline workers. Lack of training and poor supervision and support from managers leaves frontline workers feeling undervalued. Again, organisational factors are limiting the ability of frontline workers to deliver high-quality frontline care to service users. Systemic issues leading to staff absence and the loss of experienced frontline workers add to the stress experienced.

Systemic and organisational factors often exacerbate an already difficult situation for minority ethnic frontline workers and service users. Language and cultural barriers experienced by minority ethnic service users further exaggerate the barriers to good care described above. Frontline staff from these groups are also disadvantaged through discrimination in recruitment and promotion systems, and exploitation of their cultural knowledge by managers.

5 CONCLUSIONS AND RECOMMENDATIONS

This study was undertaken to review the barriers and opportunities to delivering person-centred support/care by frontline workers. This final chapter draws on the findings from this study to highlight some wider conclusions that emerge from this review. In particular, recommendations are offered for future research and for policy and practice.

Summary and conclusions

As was noted in Chapter 1, the aim of this review has been to investigate the role performed by frontline workers in delivering person-centred care to older people, disabled people and people from minority ethnic communities. To investigate this topic, a literature review and consultations with a small sample of frontline workers and service users in England and Scotland was undertaken. The thematic findings that emerged from the review and consultation have been discussed in earlier chapters. From this, three broad themes emerge, which highlight gaps or limitations in the focus taken in research to date.

First, a significant finding that emerged from this review was the limited attention within empirical research to the specific role performed by frontline workers. Most studies have focused on health and social care in relation to specific professions, e.g. social workers, domiciliary care workers, or home care workers. In so doing, attention has been given to the role of workers within a hierarchical or systemic context, focusing on both managers and frontline workers, or on service users' perceptions of the services they receive. Consequently, there is currently little empirical research that focuses specifically on the particular roles performed by, and perspectives of, those workers who are regularly performing direct care tasks, working centrally with families and service users, and working to implement an often changing policy and practice environment.

Second, this review highlights divergences in the quality of care offered within generic and specialist health or social care settings, and between statutory and voluntary sector providers. The review suggests that specialist services were regarded as of higher quality, as better resourced and as offering a wider range of supports than generic/statutory providers can deliver as a result of limits of time, resources, expertise, etc. There was also evidence that concerns about co-ordination and joint working can be overcome through the use of particular specialist workers who take a holistic perspective focusing on the person rather than on a particular service. This approach fits within a person-centred approach rather than being service driven and thus may explain the relatively positive view of these services. However, these findings do suggest a need to know more about the particular challenges facing generic care workers and how these can be overcome within their particular organisational contexts. It also suggests needing to know more about why specialist providers are perceived as offering a higher-quality service, and the extent to which this perception is based on actual differences in practice between workers or rather on higher levels of resourcing and time availability.

Third, the review suggests a constantly changing policy and practice context within which health and social care work takes place. While policy and practice change is recorded and discussed through the emergence of statutory instruments, policy documents, good-practice guidelines and critiques of policy change, there is little direct attention to the specific role of frontline workers in implementing and taking forward policy change in a practice context, nor how this impacts either positively or negatively on their ability to deliver quality care services that meet service users' needs. There are also questions as to the extent to which policy change meets service users' needs and the extent to which service users are consulted on planned policy change prior to it occurring.

It was not possible through this review to explore models of good practice in frontline health and social care given that the remit was to summarise and draw out messages from literature.

Recommendations

With the aim of this review being to explore the barriers and opportunities to delivering person-centred support/care for disabled people, older people and people from minority ethnic communities, we turn our attention here to a number of recommendations that emerge from this study. We first offer some specific research recommendations that could be undertaken to fill gaps in current knowledge. We then offer some recommendations for policy and practice that could both aid decision making and further add to knowledge on this subject.

Research recommendations

From the above themes we have identified four specific research topics that could be developed.

- A study to explore the specific roles of frontline worker(s) and the requirements of them by service users focusing on gathering views from both frontline workers and service users. This would provide an alternative and more focused approach to the previous service-delivery approach that has dominated research, while also attempting specifically to draw together a better understanding of the shared and diverging views of those who deliver services and those who receive them.

- A study that engages directly with frontline workers to explore their motivations, satisfactions and frustrations in their role – in particular, focusing directly on the drivers and challenges facing frontline workers. It could also investigate the diversity of frontline workers, relating to the tasks they undertake within their role and their age, gender and ethnicity.

- Research is required to gather a richer picture of service users' views and experiences of frontline care and support. A more detailed picture is needed of the potential divergences between different service users' requirements, which could help better understand the complexity of delivering care and support packages in practice. This information would offer greater knowledge to frontline workers and service managers in relation to understanding the complexities of service users' requirements and recognising where there are gaps in current provision.

- A study that aims to understand how frontline workers navigate the often contradictory demands of policy and practice change and the needs of service users. This could potentially offer insights into the complexities of meeting professional requirements while also delivering a suitable care/support package to their clients.

Policy and practice recommendations

Turning now to look at the policy and practice recommendations, four areas are identified where further work could be undertaken.

- A scoping study could be undertaken to gather information on what frontline workers and service users defined as 'good-quality support'. This would improve knowledge relating to the notion of 'good-quality support' while also focusing more directly on gathering the views of service users and frontline workers rather than managers and policy makers.

- A national mapping exercise could be undertaken to identify and record both innovative and best practice where these were taking place. This would not only offer an opportunity to disseminate this information, but would also encourage and promote quality frontline care and support.

- With this study finding that staff support and development were areas of particular need for frontline workers, more needs to be known about the role played by training in meeting staff need – in particular, how training might complement or take into account staff characteristics, qualities and skills. A consultation exercise with frontline workers on their training needs and how these could best be met may offer one way of gathering knowledge of this issue.

- Finally, with practice lagging well behind policy rhetoric and ideology, consultation with those at the grass roots (frontline workers, service users and voluntary sector organisations) could shed some light on the reason for the delays occurring in practice. It could also offer suggestions from the grass-roots perspective for how best to implement change. The voice of service users and frontline workers could also usefully be brought into policy discourse through this exercise.

REFERENCES

ADSW (Association of Directors of Social Work) (2004) *Supporting Front Line Staff Initiative*. Edinburgh: ADSW

Aronson, J. and Neysmith, S. (1996) '"You're not just in there to do the work": depersonalizing policies and the exploitation of home care workers' labor', *Gender and Society*, Vol. 10, pp. 59–77

Audit Commission (2002) *Recruitment and Retention: A Public Service Workforce for the Twenty-first Century*. London: Audit Commission

Audit Commission (2003) *Services for Disabled Children.* London: Audit Commission

Begum, N. (1995) *Care Management and Assessment from an Anti-racist Perspective*. York: Joseph Rowntree Foundation. Available at: www.jrf.org.uk/knowledge/findings/socialcare/pdf/sc65.pdf (accessed June 2004)

Beresford, P. (1995) *The Needs of Disabled Children and Their Families.* York: Joseph Rowntree Foundation

Beresford, P. (2003) 'The social care workforce: research issues for service users', in Social Care Workforce Research Unit *Social Care Workforce Research: Needs and Priorities*. London: King's College

Bignall, T. and Butt, J. (2000) *Between Ambition and Achievement: Young Black Disabled People's Views and Experiences of Independence and Independent Living*. York: Joseph Rowntree Foundation

Blakemore, K. (1999) 'Health and social care needs in minority communities: an over-problematized issue?', *Health and Social Care in the Community*, Vol. 8, pp. 22–30

Boehm, A. and Staples, L. (2002) 'The functions of the social worker in empowering: the voices of consumers and professionals', *Social Work*, Vol. 47, pp. 449–59

Bond, J., Farrow, G., Gregson, B., Bamford, C., Buck, D., McNamee, P. and Wright, K. (1999) 'Informal caregiving for frail older people at home and in long term care institutions: who are the key supporters?', *Health and Social Care in the Community*, Vol. 7, No. 6, pp. 434–44

Bowes, A. and Dar, N. (2000a) *Family Support and Community Care: A Study of South Asian Older People.* Edinburgh: Scottish Executive Central Research Unit

Bowes, A. and Dar, N. (2000b) 'Researching social care for minority ethnic older people: implications of some Scottish research', *British Journal of Social Work*, Vol. 30, pp. 305–21

Bowes, A. and Wilkinson, H. (2003) 'We didn't know it would get that bad: South Asian experiences of dementia and the services response', *Health and Social Care in the Community*, Vol. 11, pp. 387–96

Brooker, D. (2004) 'What is person-centred care in dementia?', *Reviews in Clinical Gerontology*, Vol. 13, pp. 215–22

Bryan, K., Axelrod, L., Maxim, L., Bell, L. and Jordan, L. (2002) 'Working with older people with communication difficulties: an evaluation of care worker training', *Aging and Mental Health*, Vol. 6, pp. 248–54

Buchan, J., Jobanputra, R. and Gough, P. (2004) *London Calling? The International Recruitment of Health Workers to the Capital.* London: King's Fund

Butt, J. and O'Neil, A. (2004) *Let's Move on: Black and Minority Ethnic Older People's Views on Research Findings.* York: Joseph Rowntree Foundation

Cambridge, P. and McCarthy, M. (2001) 'User focus groups and Best Value in services for people with learning disabilities', *Health and Social Care in the Community*, Vol. 9, No. 6, pp. 476–89

Carmichael, A. and Brown, L. (2002) 'The future challenge of direct payments', *Disability and Society*, Vol. 17, pp. 797–808

Chambo, R. and Ahmed, W. (2000) 'Language, communication and information: the needs of parents caring for a severely disabled child', in W. Ahmed (ed.) *Ethnicity, Disability and Chronic Illness.* Buckingham: Open University Press

Chan, T. and Cheung, T. (2004) *Central Scotland Chinese Association: Community Survey Report.* Stirling: Central Scotland Chinese Association

Chevannes, M. (2002) 'Issues in education health professionals to meet the diverse needs of patients and other service users from ethnic minority groups', *Journal of Advanced Nursing*, Vol. 39, pp. 290–8

Clark, H. and Spafford, I. (2001) *Piloting Choice and Control for Older People: An Evaluation.* Bristol: The Policy Press

Clark, H., Gough, H. and Macfarlane, A. (2004) *'It Pays Dividends': Direct Payments and Older People.* Bristol: The Policy Press

Cobban, N. (2004) 'Improving domiciliary care for people with dementia and their carers: the raising the standard project', in A. Innes, C. Archibald and C. Murphy (eds) *Dementia and Social Inclusion.* London: Jessica Kingsley

Cockerill, R., O'Brien Palla, L., Murray, M., Dorran, D., Sidani, S., Shaw, B. and Lochhaas Gerlach, J. (2002) 'Adequacy of time per visit in community nursing', *Research and Theory for Nursing Practice: An International Journal*, Vol. 16, pp. 43–51

Culley, L. (2000) 'Equal opportunities policies and nursing employment within the British National Health Service', *Journal of Advanced Nursing*, Vol. 33, pp. 130–7

Dalley, G. and Denniss, M. (2001) *Trained to Care? Investigating the Skills and Competencies of Care Assistants in Homes for Older People.* London: Centre for Policy on Ageing

Davies, S., Slack, R., Laker, S. and Philp, I. (1999) 'The educational preparation of staff in nursing homes: relationship with resident autonomy', *Journal of Advanced Nursing*, Vol. 29, pp. 208–17

Davis, A., Ellis, K. and Rummery, K. (1998) *Access to Assessment: The Perspectives of Practitioners, Disabled People and Carers.* York: Joseph Rowntree Foundation

Department of Health (2002) *Research Governance Framework for Health and Social Care.* London: The Stationery Office

Department of Health (2004) Direct Payments homepage. Available at: http://www.dh.gov.uk/PolicyAndGuidance/OrganisationPolicy/FinanceAndPlanning/DirectPayments/fs/en (accessed June 2004)

Douglas, A., MacDonald, C. and Taylor, M. (1998) *Service Users' Perspectives of 'Floating Support'.* York: Joseph Rowntree Foundation

Ellis, K., Davis, A. and Rummery, K. (1999) 'Needs assessment, street-level bureaucracy and the new community care', *Social Policy and Administration*, Vol. 33, pp. 262–80

Evans, R. and Banton, M. (2001) *Involving Black Disabled People in Shaping Services.* York: Joseph Rowntree Foundation

Finlayson, B. (2002) *Counting the Smiles: Morale and Motivation in the NHS.* London: King's Fund

Finlayson, B., Dixon. J., Meadows, S. and Blair, G. (2002) 'Mind the gap: the policy response to the NHS nursing shortage', *British Medical Journal*, Vol. 325, pp. 541–4

Ford, J., Quilgars, D. and Rugg, J. (1998) *Creating Jobs? The Employment Potential of Domiciliary Care.* Bristol: Policy Press

Foster, G. (2004) 'Managing front line practice: women and men: the social care workforce', in D. Statham (ed.) *Managing Front Line Practice in Social Care.* London: Jessica Kingsley

Francis, J. and Netten, A. (2004) 'Raising the quality of home care: a study of service user views', *Social Policy and Administration*, Vol. 38, pp. 290–305

Gerrish, K. (2001) 'The nature and effect of communication difficulties arising from interactions between district nurses and South Asian patients and their carers', *Journal of Advanced Nursing*, Vol. 33, pp. 566–74

Gillam, S. and Levenson, R. (1999) 'Linkworkers in primary care', *British Medical Journal*, Vol. 319, p. 1215

Godfrey, A. (2000) 'What impact does training have on the care received by older people in residential homes?', *Social Work Education*, Vol. 19, pp. 55–65

Halliday, J. and Asthana, S. (2004) 'The emergent role of the link worker: a study in collaboration', *Journal of Interprofessional Care*, Vol. 18, pp.17–28

Hardy, B., Young, R. and Wistow, G. (1999) 'Dimensions of choice in the assessment and care management process: the views of older people, carers and care managers', *Health and Social Care in the Community*, Vol. 7, pp. 483–91

Harlow, E. (2004) 'Why don't women want to be social workers anymore? New managerialism, post-feminism and the shortage of social workers in Social Service Departments in England and Wales', *European Journal of Social Work*, Vol. 7, pp. 167–79

Harrison, S. and Smith, C. (2003) 'Trust and moral motivation: redundant resources in health and social care', *Policy and Politics*, Vol. 32, pp. 371–86

Hawthorne, K., Rahman, J. and Pill, R. (2003) 'Working with Bangladeshi patients in Britain: perspectives from Primary Health Care', *Family Practice*, Vol. 20, pp. 185–91

Henwood, M. (2001) *Future Imperfect? Report of the King's Fund Care and Support Inquiry.* London: King's Fund

Henwood, M. and Waddington, E. (2002) *User and Carer Messages, Outcomes of Social Care for Adults (OSCA).* Leeds: Nuffield Institute for Health, University of Leeds

Hertzberg, A. and Ekmann, S. (2000) '"We, not them and us?" Views on the relationships and interactions between staff and relatives of older people permanently living in nursing homes', *Journal of Advanced Nursing*, Vol. 31, pp. 614–22

Holborn, S.and.Vietze, P. (1999) 'Acknowledging barriers in adopting person centred planning', *Mental Retardation*, Vol. 37, pp. 117–24

Hunter, M. (2003) 'Young, gifted and stuck', *Community Care*, 24–30 July, pp. 32–4

Jacques, I. and Innes, A. (1998) 'Who cares about care assistant work?', *The Journal of Dementia Care*, November/December, pp. 33–7

Johnson, M., Cullen, L. and Patsios, D. (1999) *Managers in Long-term Care: Their Quality and Qualities.* Bristol: The Policy Press

Jones, C. (2001) 'Voices from the front line: state social workers and New Labour', *British Journal of Social Work*, Vol. 31, pp. 547–62

Jones, M. (2000) 'Hope and despair at the front line: observations on integrity and change in the human services', *International Social Work*, Vol. 43, pp. 365–80

JRF (Joseph Rowntree Foundation) (1995) *Developing User and Carer Centred Community Care.* York: Joseph Rowntree Foundation

JRF (1999) *Supporting Disabled Children and Their Families.* York: Joseph Rowntree Foundation

Kersten, P., George, S., Mclellan, L., Smith, J. and Mullee, M. (2000) 'Disabled people and professionals differ in their perceptions of rehabilitation needs', *Journal of Public Health Medicine*, Vol. 22, pp. 393–9

Kestenbaum, A. (1999) *What Price Independence? Independent Living and People with High Support Needs.* Bristol: The Policy Press

Keywood, K., Fovargue, S. and Flynn, M. (1999) *Adults with Learning Difficulties' Involvement in Health Care Decision Making.* York: Joseph Rowntree Foundation

Khanchandani, R. and Gillam, S. (1999) 'The ethnic minority linkworker: a key member of the primary health care team?', *British Journal of General Practice*, Vol. 49, pp. 993–4

Kharicha, K., Levin, E., Iliffe, S. and Davey, B. (2004) 'Social work, general practice and evidence based policy in the collaborative care of older people: current problems and future possibilities', *Health and Social Care in the Community*, Vol. 12, pp. 134–41

King's Fund (2004) *The NHS Workforce.* London: King's Fund

Lelliott, P., Beevor, A., Hogman, G., Hyslop, J., Lathlean, J. and Ward, M. (2003) 'Carers' and users' expectations of services – carer version (CUES-C): a new instrument to support the assessment of carers of people with a severe mental illness', *Journal of Mental Health*, Vol. 12, No. 2, pp. 143–52

Lindesay, J. and Skea, D. (1997) 'Gender and interactions between care staff and elderly nursing home residents with dementia', *International Journal of Geriatric Psychiatry*, Vol. 12, pp. 344–8

McCormack, B. (2004) 'Person-centredness in gerontological nursing: an overview of the literature', *International Journal of Older People Nursing*, Vol. 13, pp. 31–8

McFarlane, L. and McLean, J. (2003) 'Education and training for direct care workers', *Social Work Education*, Vol. 22, pp. 385–99

Magito-McLaughlin, D., Spinosa, T. and Marsalis, M. (2002) 'Overcoming the barriers: moving towards a service model that is conductive to Person Centred Planning', in S. Holborn and P. Vietze (eds) *Person Centred Planning: Research, Practice and Future Directions*. Baltimore, MD: Paul Brookes Publishing

Mansell, J. and Beadle-Brown, J. (2004) 'Person-centred planning or person-centred action? Policy and practice in intellectual disability services', *Journal of Applied Research in Intellectual Disabilities*, Vol. 17, pp. 1–9

Meek, I. (1998) 'Evaluation of the role of the health care assistant within a community mental health intensive care team', *Journal of Nursing Management*, Vol. 6, pp. 11–19

Menon, S., McKinlay, I. and Faragher, E. (2001) 'Knowledge and attitudes in multicultural healthcare', *Child: Care, Health and Development*, Vol. 27, pp. 439–50

Middleton, L. (1998) 'Services for disabled children: integrating the perspective of social workers', *Child and Family Social Work*, Vol. 3, pp. 239–46

Moniz-Cook, E., Millington, D. and Silver, M. (1997) 'Residential care for older people: job satisfaction and psychological health in care staff', *Health and Social Care in the Community*, Vol. 5, pp. 124–33

Moniz-Cook, E., Woods, R. and Gardiner, E. (2000) 'Staff factors associated with perception of behaviour as "challenging" in residential and nursing homes', *Aging and Mental Health*, Vol. 4, pp. 48–55

Morris, J. (1994) 'Community care or independent living?', *Critical Social Policy*, Vol. 14, pp. 24–45

Morris, J. (2002) *Moving into Adulthood: Young Disabled People Moving into Adulthood*. York: Joseph Rowntree Foundation

Mukherjee, S., Beresford, B. and Sloper, P. (1999) 'Implementing key worker services: a case study of promoting evidence-based practice', JRF research findings

National Care Standards Commission. (2004) National Care Standards Commission homepage. Available at: http://www.carestandards.org.uk (accessed June 2004)

Nemcek, M. and Sabatier, R. (2003) 'State of evaluation: community health workers', *Public Health Nursing*, Vol. 20, pp. 260–70

Parley, F. (2001) 'Person-centred outcomes improved where a person-centred model is used?', *Journal of Learning Disabilities*, Vol. 5, pp. 299–308

Patmore, C. (2001) 'Improving home care quality: an individual-centred approach', *Quality in Ageing*, Vol. 2, No. 3, pp. 15–24

Penna, S., Paylor, I. and Soothill, K. (1995) *Job Satisfaction and Dissatisfaction amongst Residential Care Workers*. York: Joseph Rowntree Foundation

Perry, M., Carpenter, I., Challis, D. and Hope, K. (2003) 'Understanding the roles of registered general nurses and care assistants in UK nursing homes', *Journal of Advanced Nursing*, Vol. 42, No. 5, pp. 497–505

Pickard, S., Jacobs, S. and Kirk, S. (2003) 'Challenging professional roles: lay carers' involvement in health care in the community', *Social Policy and Administration*, Vol. 37, pp. 82–96

Popay, J., Rogers, A. and Williams, G. (1998) 'Rationale and standards for the systematic review of qualitative literature in health service research', *Qualitative Health Research*, Vol. 8, No. 3, pp. 341–51

Prevatt Goldstein, B. (2002) 'Catch 22 – black workers' role in equal opportunities for black service users', *British Journal of Social Work*, Vol. 32, pp. 765–78

Priestley, M. (1995) 'Dropping "E's": the missing link in quality assurance for disabled people', *Critical Social Policy*, Vol. 15, pp. 7–21

Priestley, M. (1998) 'Discourse and resistance in care assessment: integrated living and community care', *British Journal of Social Work*, Vol. 28, pp. 659–73

Raynes, N., Temple, B., Glenister, C. and Coulthard, L. (2001) *Quality at Home for Older People: Involving Service Users in Defining Home Care Specification.* Bristol: The Policy Press

Reed, J., Klein, B., Cook, G. and Stanley, D. (2003) 'Quality improvement in German and UK care homes', *International Journal of Health Care Quality Assurance*, Vol. 16, pp. 248–56

Roberts, D.Y. (2002) 'Reconceptualizing case management in theory and practice: a frontline perspective', *Health Services Management Review*, Vol. 15, pp. 147–64

Rogers, J. (1990) *Caring for People: Help at the Frontline.* Buckingham: Open University Press

Rummery, K. and Glendinning, G. (2000) 'Access to services as a civil and social rights issue: the role of welfare professionals in regulating access to and commissioning services for disabled and older people under New Labour', *Social Policy and Administration*, Vol. 34, pp. 529–50

Ryan, T., Nolan, M., Enderby, P. and Reid, D. (2004) '"Part of the family": sources of job satisfaction amongst a group of community-based dementia care workers', *Health and Social Care in the Community*, Vol. 12, pp. 111–18

Scottish Executive (2000) *Draft National Care Standards.* Available at: http://www.scotland.gov.uk/consultations/social/dncs.pdf (accessed June 2004)

Scottish Executive (2002) *Research Governance Framework for Health and Community Care.* Edinburgh: The Scottish Executive

Scottish Executive. (2004a) Direct Payments Scotland home page. Available at: http://www.dpscotland.org.uk (accessed June 2004)

Scottish Executive (2004b) *Using Care Services? National Care Standards: A Guide.* Available at: http://www.scotland.gov.uk/library5/health/csns.pdf (accessed January 2004)

SCWU (Social Care Workforce Unit) (2003) *Social Care Workforce Research: Needs and Priorities.* London: SCWU, King's College

Simon, C. and Kendrick, T. (2001) 'Informal carers: the role of general practitioners and district nurses', *British Journal of General Practice*, Vol. 51, pp. 655–7

Simon, C., Kumar, S. and Kendrick, T. (2002) 'Who cares for the carers?: the district nurse perspective', *Family Practice*, Vol. 19, pp. 29–35

Simons, K. and Watson, D. (eds) (1999) *New Directions? Day Services for People with Learning Disabilities in the 1990s: A Review of the Research.* Exeter: Centre for Evidence Based Social Services, University of Exeter

Social Services Inspectorate (1998) *They Look after Their Own Don't They? Inspection of Community Care Services for Black and Ethnic Minority Older People.* London: Department of Health

Stainton, T. (2002) 'Taking rights structurally: disability, rights and social worker responses to direct payments', *British Journal of Social Work*, Vol. 32, pp. 751–63

Stalker, K. (2002) *Young Disabled People Moving into Adulthood in Scotland.* York: Joseph Rowntree Foundation

Statham, D. (2004) *Managing Front Line Practice in Social Care.* London: Jessica Kingsley

SWRDU (Social Work Research and Development Unit) (2002) *Caring for Older People at Home.* York: SWRDU, University of York

Thornley, C. (2000) 'A question of competence? Re-evaluating the roles of the nursing auxiliary and health care assistant in the NHS', *Journal of Clinical Nursing*, Vol. 19, pp. 451–8

Ungerson, C. (1999) 'Personal assistants and disabled people: an examination of a hybrid form of work and care', *Work, Employment and Society*, Vol. 13, No. 4, pp. 583–600

UNISON (2003) *Working for Local Communities.* Available at: http://www.unison.org.uk/acrobat/13507.pdf (accessed August 2004)

Vernon, A. (2002) *Users' Views of Community Care for Asian Disabled People.* Bristol: The Policy Press

Vernon, A. and Qureshi, H. (2000) 'Community care and independence: self-sufficiency or empowerment?', *Critical Social Policy*, Vol. 20, pp. 255–76

Wick, D., Coppin, R. and Payne, S. (2003) 'Teamworking in nursing homes', *Journal of Advanced Nursing*, Vol. 45, pp. 197–204

Wilson, M. (2001) 'Black women and mental health: working towards inclusive mental health services', *Feminist Review*, Vol. 68, pp. 34–51

Witcher, S., Stalker, K., Roadburgh, M. and Jones, C. (2000) *Direct Payments: The Impact on Choice and Control for Disabled People*. Edinburgh: Scottish Executive

Workman, B. (1996) 'An investigation into how health assistants perceive their role as "support workers" to the qualified staff', *Journal of Advanced Nursing*, Vol. 23, pp. 612–19

Zarb, G. and Nadash, P. (1994) *Direct Payments for Personal Assistance*. York: Joseph Rowntree Foundation

Appendix 1: Approach to Reviewing the Literature

Defining the review question/scope of the review

The primary review question was 'what are the barriers and opportunities in providing high-quality frontline care?'.

Searching for studies

Searches of a range of databases were conducted between June and October 2004, including: MEDline, ASSIA net, BIDS, Ingenta, Psychinfo, Caredata. In addition searches were conducted using specialist literature databases including: British Institute for Learning Disabilities, Tizard Centre, the King's Fund, Centre for Policy on Ageing, Joseph Rowntree Foundation and the Audit Commission. Our search was limited to a ten-year period, 1995–2004. A reference-managing database, ProCite 5, was used to hold bibliographic details of reports.

The key search terms used were:

- frontline care

- frontline worker

- care worker

- person-centred care

- care assistant

- client-centred approach

- home help

- independence

- social worker

- choice/control

- nursing assistant/auxiliary.

The above search terms were then paired with:

- older people

- minority ethnic people/group/community

- disabled people/disability

- learning difficulty/disability.

Deciding inclusion and exclusion criteria

The review was restricted to the UK, European and North American literature exploring both research looking at frontline workers' experiences and papers containing information on barriers and opportunities in providing high-quality person-centred care. Literature was selected if it included reference to the topics included in the pro forma (Appendix 2) and the key themes outlined above. The pro forma focuses on the opportunities and barriers to delivery of good-quality care. We included 100 items, with equal numbers of papers and reports included for the following groups: older people, disabled people, people from minority ethnic communities and generic literature on frontline workers to ensure a comprehensive overview of the key themes for the groups we were focusing on. Thus a purposive approach supplemented the initial systematic approach we drew upon.

Data extraction/coding

The pro forma informed the selection of data for analysis and synthesis. This involved extracting details and results of studies and storing them in one place.

Thematic analysis

The thematic analysis of the literature used the following approach.

- Quality assessment: as recommendations are based on what is included in the review, we needed to assess the 'quality' of studies. This included an assessment of the extent to which a clear account is given of methods and findings, and how these are integrated into the overall aims of particular studies.

- Synthesis of findings: this brings together the findings of all the studies reviewed in depth and a narrative that describes patterns across studies in terms of, for example, opportunities and difficulties identified and user groups involved (Popay *et al.*, 1998).

APPENDIX 2: PRO FORMA FOR THE LITERATURE REVIEW

Frontline worker/user group	
Article title	
Type of publication	
Author/s	
Date	
Country of study	
Type of publication	
Terminology/definition of frontline worker	
Pages	
Publisher	
Perspectives on care/ person-centred care	
Barriers to good care • Systemic issues • Staff issues • User issues	
Opportunities for good care • Systemic issues • Staff issues • User issues	
Perspectives of frontline workers	
Perspectives of users	

Appendix 3: Focus group schedule – frontline workers (same topics used for service user focus group)

Warm up

Welcome and introduction to project, housekeeping, expense forms, confidentiality, anonymity, consent forms.

Tape on

- Introductions.

- Start of focus group.

Person-centred care

- What does the term 'person-centred' care mean to you?

- What does good-quality care mean to you?

- What do users want from caring situations – is this different from things you have identified above?

Prompts include: choice, independence, flexibility, reliability, familiarity, friendship (relationships).

- What currently helps you achieve good-quality care?

- What stands in the way of you providing good-quality care?

Prompts include: management, training, resources, skills, personal qualities.

- What needs to change to improve care?

Qualities of frontline workers

- What do you think are good characteristics of frontline workers?

- What qualities do you think you bring to your job (strengths)?

Prompts around: gender, age and ethnicity. Prompts around: personal qualities, e.g. good listening, patience, practical skills.

- What brings you job satisfaction?

How job is valued by others

- How do you think your job is seen by other people?

Prompt distinction between: society generally, other organisations/professions, your organisations and management, carers, service users.

Challenges of working effectively with families

- What are your experiences of working with carers and families?

- What type of relationship do you have with carers/families?

- Have you experienced difficulties when working with carers/families?

Prompt on specific issues around: working with families from minority ethnic communities, younger disabled people (and family) or people with dementia.

Prompt around potential conflicts in wishes of carers and service users.

Management, training and recruitment

1 In your organisation, how much emphasis is placed on the following issues:
   - training
   - formal supervision
   - relationships with managers
   - resources.

2 What is the level of staff turnover in your organisation?
   - Reasons for leaving?
   - Recruitment issues?
   - Levels of staff absence?

Cool down

- Any final issues wish to raise before session ends?

- Thanks for participating.

- We are around to take any questions you might have after tape goes off.